L-CITRULLINE

Enhance Athletic Performance, Boost
Cardiovascular Health, and Elevate
Your Overall Wellbeing By
Unlocking the Power of L-Citrulline

SAMANTHA ZYLAR

Contents

CHAPTER ONE

Overview

An important role for the amino acid L-citrulline is played by it in a number of bodily physiological processes. Since it is a non-essential amino acid, the body can make it on its own, but it can also be acquired from diet and supplementation.

Nitric oxide, a chemical that supports general cardiovascular health by improving blood flow, relaxing blood vessels, and increasing blood flow, is produced in large part by L-citrulline.

L-Citrulline's Significance

L-citrulline has a major effect on health and well-being, which makes it important. Its possible advantages have drawn attention, especially in the areas of erectile dysfunction, cardiovascular health, and sports performance. People can improve their quality of life by using L-Citrulline if they know what its function is.

Goals And Purpose Of The Book

This book's goal is to give readers a thorough understanding of L-citrulline by going into its history, physiological roles, possible health advantages, and real-world uses. It attempts to provide a clear and easy-to-use resource for those looking to enhance their health as well as for experts working in the fields of sports, healthcare, and nutrition.

This book's scope encompasses in-depth details on the following subjects:

• L-Citrulline's metabolism and biology.

• L-citrulline's health benefits, include enhanced cardiovascular health, enhanced exercise capacity, and possible management of problems like erectile dysfunction and hypertension.

•   Safety concerns and dosage guidelines for supplementing with L-citrulline.

•   Recipes for incorporating L-Citrulline into the diet as well as dietary sources of it.

• Recent discoveries and developing patterns pertaining to L-Citrulline.

How To Utilize This Manual

This book can be an invaluable tool for readers to comprehend and make proper use of L-Citrulline. The structure of the book aims to give readers a basic understanding of L-Citrulline as well as helpful suggestions for incorporating it into everyday living. This book will function as an all-inclusive resource to assist those seeking to enhance their physical fitness, healthcare profession, or overall health in making well-informed judgments about L-Citrulline supplementation and dietary selections.

Understanding L-Citrulline In Amino Acids

The building blocks of proteins and amino acids are essential to many physiological functions carried out by the human body. One such amino acid is L-citrulline, which we will discuss here along with its importance in the larger scheme of amino acid knowledge.

How Do Amino Acids Work?

Amino acids are nitrogen, oxygen, hydrogen, and carbon atoms combined to form organic molecules. These are the fundamental structural building blocks that come together to make proteins, which are necessary for the organization, performance, and control of several biological processes. The unique molecular structure of amino acids, which consists of an amino group (-NH2), a carboxyl group (-COOH), and a variable side chain known as the R group, is what defines them. The distinctive R group is what sets one amino acid apart from another.

Commonly found in proteins are twenty typical amino acids. Based on how these amino acids function in the creation of proteins, they are divided into two main categories:

1. Essential Amino Acids: The body is unable to produce these amino acids, hence eating is the only way to get them. They consist of valine, isoleucine, and leucine among other amino acids.

2. Non-Essential Amino Acids: The body is capable of synthesizing these amino acids, hence dietary intake is not always required. Proline, arginine, and glutamine are a few non-essential amino acid examples.

Amino Acids' Function In The Body

Beyond just helping to synthesize proteins, amino acids are essential for many other bodily processes. They support a number of vital bodily functions, including:

• Protein Synthesis: A particular sequence of amino acids joins them to create polypeptide chains, which then fold into useful proteins. Enzyme production, tissue healing, and growth all depend on this mechanism.

• Enzyme Activity: Since many enzymes are proteins, certain amino acid sequences are necessary for their catalytic activity. Enzymes are in charge of accelerating the body's biochemical processes.

• Production of Neurotransmitters: Serotonin, dopamine, and glutamate are examples of amino acids that are precursors of neurotransmitters, which are essential for the transmission of nerve signals and the control of mood.

• Metabolic Pathways: Amino acids take part in a number of metabolic processes, such as the Krebs cycle (Citric acid cycle), which is essential for the synthesis of energy in cells.

• Immune System Function: The immune system and wound healing depend on certain amino acids, such as arginine.

Amino Acid Classification

Based on a number of factors, including their chemical makeup, roles in biosynthesis, and nutritional significance, amino acids can be divided into multiple groups. Amino acids are categorized using one of three primary groups:

1. Protein surfaces are frequently home to polar amino acids, which are amino acids with polar side chains. They are able to engage in various interactions, including hydrogen bonding. Serine, threonine, and asparagine are a few examples.

2. Non-Polar Amino Acids: These amino acids are buried deep within proteins and have hydrophobic side chains. They are essential for the stability and folding of proteins. Leucine, phenylalanine, and alanine are a few examples.

3. Charged Amino Acids: Positively charged (basic) and negatively charged (acidic) amino acids are two more categories for charged amino acids. Aspartic acid and glutamic acid are examples of acidic amino acids, whereas lysine, arginine, and histidine are examples of basic amino acids. These charged amino acids are necessary for ionic interactions in proteins and for the catalysis of enzymes.

As an amino acid, L-citrulline belongs in this classification scheme. It is categorized as a non-essential amino acid and contributes to the urea cycle, which aids in the body's removal of ammonia. L-citrulline is also a topic of interest in the disciplines of sports medicine and nutrition due to its potential benefits in enhancing cardiovascular health, blood flow, and athletic performance.

In summary, the chemical building blocks of the human body's biological machinery are amino acids, such as L-citrulline. Their functions go much beyond the synthesis of proteins; they are involved in many other crucial activities that uphold life and health. Comprehending the classification, roles, and specifics of amino acids is essential to understanding the complex mechanisms of the human body.

An Introduction To L-Citrulline

Describing L-Citrulline:

L-citrulline is an amino acid that occurs naturally in food and is also produced by the body. It is essential to the urea cycle, which aids in the body's removal of ammonia. Because the body can manufacture L-citrulline, it is regarded as a non-essential amino acid. However, because of its possible health advantages, it is also sold as a dietary supplement.

Natural Sources Of L-Citrulline:

Watermelon is one of the most well-known meals to contain

L-Citrulline. Cucumbers, pumpkins, and certain legumes are among the other foods that contain this amino acid. The levels in these foods might be low, though, which is why some people use supplements to achieve particular health objectives.

Forms And Supplements:

There are several ways to take L-citrulline as a dietary supplement; the most popular ones are L-citrulline and L-citrulline malate. These supplements are frequently used to enhance blood flow, reduce muscular soreness, and support athletic performance. L-citrulline supplements are widely used by athletes and fitness enthusiasts to increase nitric oxide synthesis, which can result in better exercise capacity and recuperation. But before incorporating any new supplements into your regimen, especially if you have underlying medical concerns, it is imperative that you speak with a healthcare provider.

CHAPTER TWO

Nitric Oxide And L-Citrulline

Production Of Nitric Oxide: With a variety of physiological roles, nitric oxide (NO) is an essential signaling molecule in the human body. It is essential for controlling numerous activities, including immunological reactions, neurotransmission, and blood vessel function. Its capacity to relax and widen blood arteries, improving blood flow, is one of its most notable properties.

The Function Of L-Citrulline In The Synthesis Of Nitric Oxide: L-Citrulline is an amino acid that is naturally present in some meals and is mostly synthesized in the liver of humans. It is a crucial step in the intricate production of nitric oxide. The body can change L-citrulline into L-arginine, another amino acid when we eat meals high in L-citrulline or take L-citrulline supplements. Since L-arginine is the building block for the synthesis of nitric oxide, this conversion is essential. L-arginine is transformed into nitric oxide and citrulline when the enzyme nitric oxide synthase (NOS) is present. Therefore, by making L-arginine more available, L-citrulline indirectly aids in the synthesis of nitric oxide.

Advantages Of Elevated Nitric Oxide:

1. Better Cardiovascular Health: Higher nitric oxide levels contribute to blood vessel relaxation and enlargement, which lowers blood pressure and improves blood flow. Thus, there may be a decreased chance of cardiovascular conditions including high blood pressure and atherosclerosis.

2. Enhanced Exercise Performance: Nitric oxide can enhance the delivery of oxygen and nutrients to muscles during physical activity by boosting blood flow to those muscles. Better endurance, less weariness, and possibly even better workout performance can result from this.

3. Treatment for Erectile Dysfunction: Nitric oxide is important because it helps the blood vessels in the penile tissue relax, which is necessary to get and keep an erection. To treat erectile dysfunction, drugs like sildenafil (Viagra) increase the effects of nitric oxide.

4. Cognitive performance: Since improved blood flow to the brain maintains a constant supply of oxygen and nutrients for brain cells, it can improve cognitive performance.

5. Immune Function: Nitric oxide aids in the body's defense against infections and diseases by stimulating the immune system.

6. Healing from Wounds: Nitric oxide is essential for the dilatation of blood vessels close to wounds, which facilitates the more effective delivery of nutrients and immune cells to the injured tissue, hastening the healing process.

In conclusion, L-citrulline is essential for the body's synthesis of nitric oxide, which has numerous health advantages. It is crucial for preserving general well-being since it is especially significant for cardiovascular health, exercise capacity, and other physiological processes.

Advantages Of L-Citrulline For Health

Watermelon and other foods naturally contain the amino acid L-citrulline. It provides a number of health advantages, such as:

1.   Cardiovascular   Health: By encouraging blood vessel relaxation, L-citrulline has been connected to enhanced cardiovascular function. This can improve general heart health and lower blood pressure.

2. Athletic Performance: By lowering muscle tiredness and increasing endurance, L-citrulline is thought to improve athletic performance. By helping to eliminate waste products like ammonia, it helps to postpone the onset of weariness during physical activity.

3. Erectile dysfunction: L-citrulline is a possible natural treatment for erectile dysfunction since it may assist

in increasing blood flow. Nitric oxide levels, which are essential for blood vessel relaxation and penile erections, can rise as a result of it.

4. Additional Potential Benefits: L-citrulline is being researched for its possible advantages in mending wounds, bolstering the immune system, and reducing the signs and symptoms of illnesses including sickle cell disease. It might also play a part in lessening the discomfort in the muscles and enhancing recuperation following strenuous exercise.

Before adding L-Citrulline to your daily routine, as with any supplement or health regimen, it's imperative to speak with a healthcare provider, particularly if you have underlying medical concerns or are currently taking other drugs.

The Dosage And Usage Of L-Citrulline

Suggested Dosages:

The non-essential amino acid L-citrulline has become well-known as a dietary supplement because of its possible health advantages, especially in terms of improving cardiovascular health and athletic performance. The suggested dosage of L-citrulline may change according to a person's needs, objectives, and health. The following are some broad recommendations for

L-Citrulline Dosage:

1.   Pre-Workout   Performance Enhancement: Taking 6 to 8 grams of L-Citrulline 30 minutes prior to exercise is a typical dosage for people who want to increase their exercise capacity and decrease their level of weariness. This dosage may assist in enhancing blood flow and nitric oxide levels, which could result in less soreness in the muscles and increased endurance.

2. Cardiovascular Health: To promote heart health and lower blood pressure, some people take supplements containing L-citrulline. In this

situation, it's usually advised to take a lower daily dosage of 1. 5 to 3 grams. It's crucial to speak with a medical expert before using L-citrulline for heart health.

3. Combining with Other Supplements: To maximize its benefits, L-citrulline is frequently taken in conjunction with other supplements like L-arginine or L-carnitine. Although the dosage needs to be changed appropriately, it's crucial to adhere to the product's specific instructions.

4. Individual Variability: Be aware that different people may react differently to L-Citrulline. It is

important to discover the ideal dosage for your individual needs and tolerance by progressively increasing from lesser doses at first.

Administration And Timing:

1. Pre-Workout: It is generally recommended to take L-Citrulline 30 to 60 minutes prior to working out in order to optimize its effects. When you need the amino acid most during activity, this timing enables it to be absorbed and reach peak blood levels.

2. Supplementation on a regular basis: L-citrulline is frequently taken in several doses throughout the day by

people who use it for cardiovascular health issues or other continuous needs. This may assist in keeping the bloodstream's level constant.

3. L-citrulline is a medication that can be taken with or without food. It doesn't need to be taken at a set mealtime and is usually well accepted.

Safety Points To Remember:

When taken at prescribed levels, most persons are thought to be safe when using L-citrulline. But there are a few things to be aware of regarding safety:

1. Allergies and Sensitivities: Avoid using L-citrulline if you have a known allergy to it or if you have negative responses.

2. Medication Interactions: Before using L-Citrulline, especially if you're using it for cardiovascular health, see a doctor if you're on any medications or have any underlying medical disorders. L-Citrulline may interfere with some medications.

3. L-citrulline is metabolized in the kidneys as part of renal function. It is crucial to speak with a healthcare professional before using this supplement if you have kidney problems.

4. Pregnancy and Breastfeeding: Since there is little information on the safety of L-citrulline during these times unless directed by a healthcare professional, it is best to avoid using it.

5. Consequences: Although they are usually minor and infrequent, side effects can include gastrointestinal distress such as flatulence or diarrhea. If you encounter serious side effects, stop using the product and see a doctor.

To summarize, if taken sensibly and in compliance with suggested dosages and standards, L-citrulline be capable of prove to be a beneficial dietary supplement.

Before beginning any new supplement regimen, always get medical advice, especially if you have underlying medical concerns or are taking medication.

CHAPTER THREE

L-Citrulline And Physical Activity

An amino acid called L-citrulline is important for exercise performance and has advantages for people who work out. This is a synopsis of the relationship between L-Citrulline and exercise:

1. **Increasing Endurance:** Research has been done on the possibility that L-citrulline can increase endurance when engaging in aerobic exercises. It accomplishes this by boosting the synthesis of nitric oxide, which enhances blood flow and oxygen supply to muscles. Thus, longer periods of higher-intensity performance are possible for athletes and fitness enthusiasts, especially in long-distance running and cycling.

2. Minimizing Muscle Weariness:

L-citrulline can help lessen muscle weariness by increasing blood flow and lowering the amount of ammonia that builds up in the muscles. It may postpone the onset of muscular fatigue by encouraging improved nutrition supply and waste product elimination. Exercises like weightlifting and high-intensity interval training that need repetitive contractions may benefit most from this.

3. Use Of Pre-Workout Supplements: L-Citrulline is a popular pre-workout supplement among athletes and those who want to maximize their exercise performance. Because of the aforementioned advantages, it's frequently added to different pre-workout formulas, allowing users to train longer and harder. This amino acid can be taken as a powder or as a capsule prior to working out and is generally well-tolerated.

To sum up, L-Citrulline is a well-liked option for people looking to perform better during exercise because of its acknowledged ability to increase endurance, lessen muscle tiredness, and function as a useful component of pre-workout supplements. To make sure a supplement fits your unique health and fitness goals, you should always speak with a healthcare provider before incorporating any new ones into your routine.

Because of its possible advantages for a number of human health issues, the non-essential amino acid L-citrulline has drawn a lot of interest from scientists and proponents of health supplements. Let's explore the idea of L-Citrulline research and studies, covering current research trends and its possibilities in the future.

Research In Science On L-Citrulline:

Numerous scientific investigations have been carried out to examine the advantages and effects of L-citrulline over time. Among the well-known fields of study are:

1. Cardiovascular Health: Studies have indicated that L-Citrulline may be beneficial for heart health. It is a precursor to the chemical nitric oxide (NO), which dilates and relaxes blood vessels in an attempt to increase blood flow and possibly lower blood pressure. Investigations on its possible application for diseases like hypertension have resulted from this.

2. Exercise Performance: Because L-Citrulline has the ability to lessen muscle tiredness and improve exercise performance, it has become

more and more well-known in the fitness and sports industries. Research has examined its potential to lessen stiffness in the muscles and boost stamina when engaging in physical activities.

3. L-Citrulline is also being investigated as a potential natural treatment for erectile dysfunction. According to certain research, it might strengthen sexual function and increase blood flow to the vaginal region.

4. Ammonia Detoxification: L-citrulline is essential to the urea cycle, which aids in the body's removal of the poisonous chemical ammonia.

Because of this, it may be used as a treatment for illnesses linked to ammonia poisoning.

Trends In Current Research:

The state of L-citrulline research is always changing, and some of the current developments are as follows:

1. Combination Therapies: Scientists are looking at how L-Citrulline works in concert with other substances like L-arginine or antioxidants. These mixtures might increase their efficacy for particular medical issues.

2. Precision medicine is gaining traction by customizing L-Citrulline nutrition to each person's distinct physiology and health requirements. Customized strategies are being investigated to optimize its advantages and minimize any possible drawbacks.

3. Targeted Applications: New research is focusing on the potential uses of L-Citrulline, such as treating neurological illnesses, promoting wound healing, or lessening the consequences of some chronic illnesses.

Prospective Future:

L-citrulline research has a bright future ahead of it, with several interesting areas of study:

1. Clinical therapy: Cardiovascular diseases, neurological disorders, and metabolic syndrome are only a few of the problems for which L-citrulline may find use in clinical therapy. Its therapeutic efficacy will probably be investigated in more detail.

2. Aging and Longevity: L-citrulline has generated interest in its potential to support healthy aging and extend longevity due to its role in enhancing

blood flow and possibly lowering oxidative stress.

3. Nutraceutical Development: As the amount of data demonstrating the health advantages of L-Citrulline increases, more nutraceutical products containing this amino acid are anticipated to be developed, providing consumers with additional alternatives for supplementing their diets.

In summary, there is a growing body of evidence indicating that L-citrulline may have benefits for a variety of human health issues, and the supplement is the focus of active and varied research. It's an intriguing topic of research in the world of health and nutrition, and as it continues to develop, we may anticipate learning more about its applications and therapeutic purposes.

Including L-Citrulline In Your Daily Diet

Dietary Selections:

1. Whole Foods: Consume foods high in L-citrulline, such as watermelon, cucumbers, and pumpkins, to naturally incorporate this amino acid.

2. Balanced Diet: To provide your body with the vital nutrients it needs, make sure your diet is well-rounded

and contains a range of fruits and vegetables.

Selection Of Supplements:

1. Speak with a Healthcare Professional: Prior to taking L-citrulline supplements, speak with a healthcare professional to establish the proper dosage and make sure the supplement is appropriate for your needs and health.

2. Purity and Quality: To guarantee safety and efficacy, use reputed brands and premium supplements.

3. Dosage: Adhere to the dosage recommendations provided by your healthcare provider or on the product label.

Living Suggestions:

1. Hydration: Drink plenty of water because L-citrulline may cause an increase in urine production, which can cause dehydration.

2. Exercise: L-citrulline is frequently taken as a supplement prior to exercise. If you exercise regularly, you might be able to improve your performance by taking it before.

3. Consistency: Using L-Citrulline consistently, whether through diet or pills, is crucial for potential benefits.

4. Watch Your Health: Pay attention to how L-Citrulline affects your body and get medical advice if you feel any negative side effects.

Including L-Citrulline in your diet may improve your health in relation to circulation and physical activity, but you should take caution and pay attention to your specific needs when doing so.

CHAPTER FOUR

Possible Adverse Reactions And Safety Measures

L-citrulline is an amino acid that can be obtained as a dietary supplement or naturally occurring in some foods. It is frequently used to enhance cardiovascular health, reduce muscular soreness, and enhance sports performance.

L-citrulline, like any dietary supplement or prescription drug, may have adverse effects, so people should be cautious.

Frequent Adverse Events:

1. Gastrointestinal Distress: Taking supplements containing L-citrulline may cause moderate gastrointestinal distress in certain people. This may involve signs and symptoms like diarrhea, gas, and bloating. One possible solution to these problems could be to lower the dosage or take the supplement with food.

2. Allergic Reactions: Although they are uncommon, L-citrulline allergies can happen. An allergic reaction may manifest as hives, swelling, itching, dyspnea, and vertigo. If you have any

of these side effects after taking L-citrulline, get help right away.

3. Low Blood Pressure: It is well known that L-Citrulline helps to relax blood vessels, which can lower blood pressure. While L-Citrulline may be helpful for people with hypertension, people with low blood pressure should use caution when taking it since it may make their situation worse.

Reactions And Cautionary Notes:

1. Drug Interactions: L-citrulline may have interactions with several medications, especially those used for

hypertension and erectile dysfunction (such as sildenafil or tadalafil). When L-Citrulline is taken with these drugs, the blood pressure may decrease too much.

2. Renal Impairment: Since the kidneys are where L-citrulline is mainly processed, people who have renal problems should take caution when using this supplement. In these kinds of situations, it is best to speak with a healthcare provider to figure out the right dosage.

3. Pregnancy and Breastfeeding: Pregnant and nursing women are advised not to use L-Citrulline unless prescribed by a healthcare

professional due to the paucity of research on the supplement's safety during these times.

Who Should Avoid It?

1. Allergic Reactions: L-citrulline users with a history of allergies should refrain from using it in any form.

2. Low Blood Pressure: Since L-Citrulline supplementation can further lower blood pressure, people with hypotension (chronically low blood pressure) should exercise caution while contemplating it.

3. Medical Conditions: Before using L-Citrulline, it is important to speak with a healthcare provider if you have a medical condition or are on any medications, especially ones that influence renal function or blood pressure.

4. Pregnancy and nursing: As previously indicated, due to insufficient safety data in these groups, pregnant and nursing women should generally avoid L-Citrulline unless specifically suggested by a healthcare provider.

It's critical to keep in mind that different people may react differently to supplements. It is best to speak with a healthcare professional before beginning or stopping any supplement, including L-citrulline, as they can offer you individualized advice and keep an eye out for any possible interactions or side effects depending on your unique needs and health state.

Conclusion

In conclusion, L-citrulline is an essential amino acid that is involved in a number of physiological functions, such as the body's detoxification of ammonia and synthesis of nitric oxide. It has drawn interest due to its possible health advantages, especially in enhancing general well-being, exercise capacity, and cardiovascular health.

Summary Of The Main Points:

1. One amino acid that is found in some foods naturally is called L-citrulline. It is also available as a dietary supplement.

2. It is a precursor to nitric oxide, which promotes cardiovascular health by improving blood flow, relaxing blood vessels, and improving circulation.

3. By assisting in the elimination of ammonia from muscles, L-citrulline may improve endurance, lessen muscular pain, and improve exercise performance.

4. L-citrulline appears to have a bright future ahead of it, as research continues to examine its possible uses in conditions like erectile dysfunction, hypertension, and overall health enhancement.

Taking Charge Of Your Health With Information:

It's crucial to keep up with the most recent L-Citrulline research and scientific advancements if you want to use knowledge to improve your health.

To find out how to best incorporate L-Citrulline into your routine for health and wellness, consult with nutritionists and healthcare specialists. Recall that the keys to maximizing your well-being include a healthy diet, consistent exercise, and a holistic outlook on wellness.

A healthcare professional should always be consulted before beginning a new supplement or making big changes to your daily routine.

www.ingramcontent.com/pod-product-compliance
Lightning Source LLC
Chambersburg PA
CBHW060841260726
48661CB00002B/541